95 Juice and Meal Recipes to Treat Your Sore Throat Fast:

Naturally Cure Your Sore Throat by Eating Vitamin-Rich Foods

By

Joe Correa CSN

COPYRIGHT

This publication is designed to provide accurate and authoritative information in regard to the subject matter covered. It is sold with the understanding that neither the author nor the publisher is engaged in rendering medical advice. If medical advice or assistance is needed, consult with a doctor. This book is considered a guide and should not be used in any way detrimental to your health. Consult with a physician before starting this nutritional plan to make sure it's right for you.

ACKNOWLEDGEMENTS

This book is dedicated to my friends and family that have had mild or serious illnesses so that you may find a solution and make the necessary changes in your life.

95 Juice and Meal Recipes to Treat Your Sore Throat Fast:

Naturally Cure Your Sore Throat by Eating Vitamin-Rich Foods

By

Joe Correa CSN

CONTENTS

ABOUT THE AUTHOR

After years of Research, I honestly believe in the positive effects that proper nutrition can have over the body and mind. My knowledge and experience has helped me live healthier throughout the years and which I have shared with family and friends. The more you know about eating and drinking healthier, the sooner you will want to change your life and eating habits.

Nutrition is a key part in the process of being healthy and living longer so get started today. The first step is the most important and the most significant.

INTRODUCTION

95 Juice and Meal Recipes to Treat Your Sore Throat Fast: Naturally Cure Your Sore Throat by Eating Vitamin-Rich Foods

By Joe Correa CSN

Having a sore throat is an uncomfortable condition followed by irritation and swallowing difficulties.

Building your immune system through a variety of vitamin-rich foods is always the best way to fight off different viruses that cause a sore throat and other illnesses. Most of us know this theoretically, but we don't seem to notice how important what we eat can be towards our recovery. We ignore or even completely avoid some basic nutritional guidelines, and fall into a trap and end up curing the condition instead of preventing it. This condition is not dangerous unless it lasts for an extended period of time and that's when you need to visit a doctor.

When dealing with a sore throat, eating can become painful but you need to eat to get better. That's why I wanted to share with you some basic tips on what to eat until you get better.

The first rule of nutrition, when it comes to a sore throat, is to eat soft or cooked food. This doesn't come as a surprise. However, I wanted to share with you some amazingly tasty recipes that require very little chewing, and are perfectly healthy at the same time. I believe that is the greatest challenge when you have a sore throat.

These delicious recipes will ease your swallowing difficulties and you'll enjoy every single bite.

Also, I wanted to go one step forward with these recipes and give you the best possible collection of nutrients you can find to boost your immune system and prevent this condition from happening often.

A sore throat can be extremely irritating and can drain all your energy. Let this book serve as your health guide and help you finally forget about this common winter condition.

COMMITMENT

In order to improve my condition, I *(your name)*, commit to eating more of these foods on a daily basis and to exercise at least 30 minutes daily:

- Berries (especially blueberries), peaches, cherries, apples, apricots, oranges, lemon juice, grapefruit, tangerines, mandarins, pears, etc.
- Broccoli, spinach, collard greens, sweet potatoes, avocado, artichoke, baby corn, carrots, celery, cauliflower, onions, etc.
- Whole grains, steel-cut oats, oatmeal, quinoa, barley, etc.
- Black beans, red bean beans, garbanzo beans, lentils, etc.
- Nuts and seeds including: walnuts, cashews, flaxseeds, sesame seeds, etc.
- Fish
- 8 – 10 glasses of water

Sign here

X_____

95 JUICE AND MEAL RECIPES TO TREAT YOUR SORE THROAT FAST: NATURALLY CURE YOUR SORE THROAT BY EATING VITAMIN-RICH FOODS

MEAL RECIPES

1.   Lemony Chicken Soup

Ingredients:

2 lbs of chicken breasts, cut into bite-sized pieces

1 large carrot, sliced

½ cup of celery, chopped

¼ cup of spring onions, chopped

3 tbsp of lemon juice, freshly squeezed

2 large eggs

4 tbsp of olive oil

¼ tsp of salt

¼ tsp of black pepper, ground

Preparation:

Preheat the oil in a large nonstick saucepan over a medium-high temperature. Add carrot, celery, and onions and cook for 5 minutes, stirring constantly. Now, add chicken and cook for another 5 minutes, or until chicken is slightly browned. Pour enough water to cover all ingredients and bring it to a boil. Reduce the heat to low and cover with a lid. Add more water to adjust the thickness of the soup. Simmer for about 30-40 minutes.

Meanwhile, combine eggs and lemon juice in a medium bowl. Sprinkle with some salt and pepper and pour into the saucepan. Stir well and let it cook for 5 minutes, or until eggs are set. Remove from the heat and serve warm.

Nutrition information per serving: Kcal: 401, Protein: 46.2g, Carbs: 2.1g, Fats: 22.3g

2.   Homemade Spicey Polenta

Ingredients:

1 lb of corn flour

4 cups of water

5 tbsp of olive oil

1 cup of Greek yogurt

½ tsp of Cayenne pepper

1 tbsp of butter

¼ tsp of salt

Preparation:

Pour the water into a deep pot and bring it to a boil.

Add olive oil and salt and reduce the heat to medium. Slowly stir in the corn flour. Cook until the mixture thickens, stirring constantly. Remove from the heat and let it cool for a while. Top with yogurt and set aside.

Meanwhile, melt the butter in a frying pan over a medium high temperature. stir in cayenne pepper and cook for 1 minute. Remove from the heat sprinkle the polenta with this mixture.

Nutrition information per serving: Kcal: 209, Protein: 6.2g, Carbs: 44.5g, Fats: 12.8g

3.   Strawberry Melon Milkshake

Ingredients:

½ cup of fresh strawberries

½ large banana, chopped

1 cup of melon, chopped

3 tbsp of lemon juice, freshly squeezed

¼ tsp of cinnamon, ground

2 cups of skim milk

Preparation:

Combine all ingredients in a food processor and blend until nicely smooth. Transfer to a serving glasses and serve immediately.

Nutrition information per serving: Kcal: 82, Protein: 4.7g, Carbs: 14.8g, Fats: 0.3g

4.   Tomato-Bean Soup

Ingredients:

2 lbs of medium-sized tomatoes, diced

1 cup of white beans, pre-cooked

1 small onion, diced

2 garlic cloves, crushed

1 cup of heavy cream

4 tbsp of skim milk

1 cup of vegetable broth

2 tbsp of fresh parsley, finely chopped

¼ tsp of black pepper, ground

2 tbsp of olive oil

½ tsp of salt

Preparation:

Place the beans in a pot of boiling water and cook until soften. Remove from the heat and drain well. Set aside.

Preheat the oil in a large saucepan over a medium-high temperature. Add onions and garlic and stir-fry for 5 minutes, or until translucent. Stir in the tomatoes, white beans, parsley, and salt. Add milk to balance the bitterness. Stir once, then add vegetable broth. Reduce the heat to low and cook for 45 minutes and then remove from the heat.

Stir in sour cream and serve.

Nutrition information per serving: Kcal: 317, Protein: 12.8g, Carbs: 34.9g, Fats: 15.5g

5. Blueberry Pancakes with Almond Cream

Ingredients:

4 tbsp of flaxseeds

12 tbsp of water

4 tbsp buckwheat flour

1 cup of almond milk

¼ tsp of salt

1 cup of almond cream

1 cup of fresh blueberries

Flaxseed oil

Preparation:

Combine flaxseeds with ½ cup of water and set aside to soak.

Meanwhile, combine other ingredients in a bowl and add flax seed mixture. Beat well with an electric mixer on high speed.

Heat up the oil in a skillet over a medium-high temperature. Pour some of the mixture in the skillet and fry the pancakes for about 2-3 minutes, on each side. This mixture should give you about 8 pancakes.

Top each pancake with almond cream and fresh blueberries. Serve.

Nutrition information per serving: Kcal: 358, Protein: 8.9g, Carbs: 20.9g, Fats: 28.7g

6.   Fresh Lettuce with Vinegar & Lime

Ingredients:

4 oz of fresh lettuce, chopped

¼ cup of apple cider vinegar

3 tbsp of fresh lemon juice

2 tsp of honey

2 garlic cloves, crushed

¼ cup of extra-virgin olive oil

2 tbsp of fresh lime juice

Preparation:

Combine the vinegar, lemon juice, honey, garlic, olive oil, and lime juice in a jar. Seal the lid and shake until well combined. Let it stand for at least 20 minutes to allow flavors to mingle.

Place the lettuce in a large bowl and drizzle with the dressing. Toss to coat and serve.

Nutrition information per serving: Kcal: 265, Protein: 0.7g, Carbs: 10.4g, Fats: 25.5g

7.   Mashed Sweet Potatoes with Onions

Ingredients:

3 cups of sweet potatoes, pre-cooked

1 cup of spring onions, finely chopped

1 small red onion, chopped

1 tbsp of lemon juice

1 tbsp of olive oil

½ tsp of salt

¼ tsp of black pepper, ground

Preparation:

Place the potatoes in a pot of boiling water. Cook until fork-tender. Remove from the heat and drain well. Set aside to cool for a while.

Transfer the potatoes to a food processor. Add a pinch of salt and pepper and process until nicely pureed. Transfer the mixture to a large bowl. Stir in the spring onions, red onion and drizzle with lemon juice and olive oil. Season with some extra salt and pepper to taste.

Serve cold.

Nutrition information per serving: Kcal: 218, Protein: 3.2g Carbs: 46.7g Fats: 5.1g

8.   Quinoa & Beans Porridge

Ingredients:

1 cup of white quinoa, pre-cooked

1 cup of white beans, pre-cooked

½ cup of fresh parsley

1 small onion, finely chopped

2 garlic cloves, minced

1 cup of button mushrooms, sliced

¼ tsp of salt

4 tbsp of olive oil

¼ tsp of black pepper, ground

Preparation:

Place quinoa in a deep pot and add 3 cups of water. Bring it to a boil and then reduce the heat to low. Cover with a lid and cook for 15 minutes. Remove from the heat and fluff with a fork. Set aside.

Place the beans in a pot of boiling water and cook until soften. Remove from the heat and drain well. Set aside.

Preheat the oil in a large skillet over a medium-high temperature. Add chopped onion and garlic. Stir-fry for 5 minutes, or until translucent.

Add cooked quinoa, white beans, parsley, button mushrooms, and 2 cups of water. Mix well and cook for 15 minutes, or until the liquid evaporates. Remove from the heat and transfer to a bowl. Sprinkle with pepper and mix well. Serve warm.

Nutrition information per serving: Kcal: 619, Protein: 25.2g, Carbs: 82.0g, Fats: 22.9g

9.   Kale Smoothie

Ingredients:

1 cup of almond milk

1 cup of fresh kale, finely chopped

½ peach, sliced

1 cup of melon

1 tsp of turmeric, ground

1 tbsp of sesame seeds

1 tsp of honey

Preparation:

Place the ingredients in a food processor. Pulse to combine and transfer to a serving glasses. Refrigerate for 30 minutes before serving.

Nutrition information per serving: Kcal: 249, Protein: 3.8g, Carbs: 16.4g, Fats: 20.8g

10.   Brown Rice with Stewed Vegetables

Ingredients:

1 cup of brown rice, uncooked

8 oz of fresh cauliflower

2 medium-sized carrots, sliced

1 medium-sized celery root, sliced

3 tbsp of butter

1 tsp of sea salt

½ tsp of black pepper, ground

Preparation:

Place the rice in a deep pot. Add about 3 cups of water and bring it to a boil. Reduce the heat and continue to cook until the liquid evaporates. Remove from the heat and set aside.

Meanwhile, place the vegetables in a pot of boiling water and cook until soft. Remove from the heat and drain.

Melt the butter in a large saucepan over a medium-high temperature. Add cooked rice, salt, pepper and stir-fry for 3-4 minutes. Mix well and serve with sliced vegetables.

Nutrition information per serving: Kcal: 427, Protein: 6.7g, Carbs: 56.7g, Fats: 20.5g

11.   Sour Cabbage Salad

Ingredients:

4 oz fresh cabbage, thinly shredded

¼ cup apple cider vinegar

¼ tsp of salt

¼ tsp of black pepper, ground

Preparation:

In a small saucepan, combine apple cider vinegar, pepper, and salt and bring it to a boil. Stir well once and remove from the heat.

Pour this warm dressing over cabbage and toss well to combine. Serve immediately.

Nutrition information per serving: Kcal: 175, Protein: 1.5g, Carbs: 7.5g, Fats: 0.1g

12.   Gorgonzola Soup

Ingredients:

10 oz of Gorgonzola cheese, crumbled

1 cup of broccoli, finely chopped

1 tbsp of olive oil

½ cup of skim milk

½ cup of vegetable broth

1 tbsp of parsley, finely chopped

½ tsp of salt

¼ tsp of black pepper, ground

Preparation:

Preheat the oil in a deep pot over a medium-high temperature. Add broccoli and parsley and sprinkle with salt and pepper. Add 2 tablespoons of water to prevent sticking to the pot. Cook for 5 minutes, stirring constantly.

Now, add cheese, vegetable broth and milk. Add water to adjust the thickness of the soup. Stir well and bring it to a boil. Reduce the heat to low and cover with a lid. Cook for 30 minutes and remove from the heat.

Nutrition information per serving: Kcal: 397, Protein: 23.7g, Carbs: 10.3g, Fats: 31.6g

13. Green Bean Puree

Ingredients:

8 oz of fresh green beans

1 cup of Greek yogurt

½ tsp of salt

2 tbsp of olive oil

¼ tsp of black pepper, ground

Preparation:

Clean the beans and place in a steamer. Cook for 5 minutes, or until soften.

Remove from the heat and rinse well under the cold water. Place in a food processor and add Greek yogurt, oil, and salt. Blend well until smooth mixture and transfer to a serving bowl. Season with some pepper and serve.

Nutrition information per serving: Kcal: 113, Protein: 5.7g, Carbs: 6.0g, Fats: 8.0g

14. Fig Fruit Salad with Chia Seeds

Ingredients:

2 medium-sized plums, sliced

2 medium-sized figs, sliced

½ Alkmene apple, chopped into bite-sized pieces

1 tbsp of chia seeds

2 tbsp of fig jam

Preparation:

Place apple chops, plums and figs in a pot of boiling water. Cook for 2 minutes and remove from the heat. Drain well and set aside to cool.

Transfer the apples and plums to a food processor, and place figs in a medium bowl. Blend for 30 seconds and transfer to a bowl with figs.

Stir in the fig jam and toss to combine. Top with chia seeds. Serve cold.

Nutrition information per serving: Kcal: 178, Protein: 2.3g, Carbs: 34.6g, Fats: 2.5g

15. Avocado Puree

Ingredients:

2 ripe avocados, pitted and diced

3 organic limes, juiced

2 tbsp of extra-virgin olive oil

1 garlic clove, crushed

2 tbsp of fresh cilantro, minced

½ tsp of salt

¼ tsp of black pepper, ground

Preparation:

Combine the ingredients in a food processor. Cover and puree until nicely smooth. Refrigerate or serve immediately.

Nutrition information per serving: Kcal: 355, Protein: 2.6g, Carbs: 12.0g, Fats: 35.5g

16.   Fresh Apple & Figs Smoothie

Ingredients:

1 small green apple, sliced

4 fresh figs, halved

1 small kiwi, peeled and sliced

¼ cup of spinach, finely chopped

¼ cup of lime

1 tsp of honey

½ cup of rice milk

½ cup of water

Preparation:

Combine all ingredients in a food processor and blend until nicely smooth. Transfer to a serving glasses and refrigerate before serving.

Nutrition information per serving: Kcal: 150, Protein: 1.8g, Carbs: 37.7g, Fats: 0.9g

17.   Broccoli Soup

Ingredients:

2 oz of fresh broccoli, chopped

2 oz Brussel sprouts, chopped

¼ cup of fresh parsley, finely chopped

1 tsp of dried thyme, ground

1 tbsp of lemon juice, freshly squeezed

¼ tsp of sea salt

Preparation:

Place the broccoli in a deep pot and pour enough water to cover. Bring it to a boil and cook until tender. Remove from the heat and drain.

Transfer to a food processor. Add fresh parsley, thyme, and about 1 cup of water. Pulse until smooth mixture. Return to a pot and add some more water. Bring it to a boil and cook for several minutes, over a minimum temperature. Season with salt and add fresh lemon juice. Serve warm.

Nutrition information per serving: Kcal: 146, Protein: 4.2g, Carbs: 10.8g, Fats: 0.7g

18.   Brown Rice Mushroom Risotto

Ingredients:

1 cup of brown rice

1 cup of button mushrooms, sliced

½ medium-sized onion, finely chopped

3 spring onions, sliced

3 tbsp of extra-virgin olive oil

½ tsp of salt

1 tsp of dry marjoram, crushed

Preparation:

Place the rice in a deep pot. Add 2 cups of water and bring it to a boil. Reduce the heat and cook until the water evaporates. Stir occasionally. Set aside.

Heat up one tablespoon of olive oil over a medium-high heat. Add chopped onion and stir-fry for 3-4 minutes, stirring constantly. Now add the mushrooms and continue to cook until the water evaporates.

Stir in the remaining olive oil, rice, spring onions, salt, and marjoram. Add one cup of water and continue to cook for another 10 minutes.

Serve warm.

Nutrition information per serving: Kcal: 550, Protein: 9.0g, Carbs: 77.9g, Fats: 23.7g

19.   Chocolate Pudding

Ingredients:

2 cups of almond milk

1 tbsp of walnuts, finely chopped

1 tbsp of hazelnuts, finely chopped

2 tsp of cocoa powder, raw

1 tsp of cinnamon, ground

½ tbsp of vanilla extract

1 tsp of honey, raw

Preparation:

In a medium-sized saucepan, bring 2 cups of almond milk to boil. Add nuts, cocoa, honey, vanilla extract, and stir well. Cook for about 10 minutes, or until you get a creamy mixture. Stir in some cinnamon and remove from the heat. Allow it to cool in the refrigerator before serving.

Nutrition information per serving: Kcal: 412, Protein: 4.8g, Carbs: 12.8g, Fats: 40.8g

20. Eggplant Stew

Ingredients:

4 medium-sized eggplants, chopped

3 large tomatoes, finely chopped

2 red bell peppers, finely chopped

¼ cup of tomato paste

¼ cup of fresh parsley, finely chopped

2 tbsp of salted capers, rinsed and drained

¼ cup of olive oil

1 tsp of sea salt

Preparation:

Place the chopped eggplant in a pot of boiling water and cook until soften. Remove from the heat and drain well. Set aside to cool for a while. Transfer the eggplant to a food processor and blend until pureed. Set aside.

Grease the bottom of a deep pot with oil. Add tomatoes, peppers, capers, and tomato paste. Pour the eggplant puree and add water enough to cover all ingredients. Bring it to a boil and reduce the heat to low. Cover with a lid and add more water if needed. Sprinkle with salt and pepper to taste and cook for 1 hour. Remove from the heat and serve with yogurt or sour cream. However, this is optional.

Nutrition information per serving: Kcal: 122, Protein: 3.2g, Carbs: 18.2g, Fats: 5.7g

21. Brown Rice Pudding with Raspberries and Chia Seeds

Ingredients:

¾ cup of brown rice

1 cup of rice milk

¼ cup of honey

1 tbsp of almond butter

¼ tsp of salt

½ cup of raspberries

¼ cup of walnuts

2 tbsp of chia seeds

Preparation:

Bring 2 cups of water to a boil. Add rice and reduce the heat. Cover and cook for about 15 minutes.

Now add one cup of rice milk, honey, almond butter, and salt. Continue to cook for five more minutes. Remove from the heat and cool for a while.

Top with fresh raspberries, walnuts, and chia seeds. Serve.

Nutrition information per serving: Kcal: 232, Protein: 7.7g, Carbs: 76.2g, Fats: 11.6g

22.   Cold Green Bean Salad with Garlic

Ingredients:

1 lb of green beans, trimmed

¼ cup of extra-virgin olive oil

1 tbsp of Dijon mustard

2 garlic cloves, crushed

1 tbsp of lime juice

Preparation:

Boil a pot of water and add one teaspoon of salt and green beans. Cook until tender. This should take about 10-15 minutes. Rinse and drain.

Meanwhile, combine the crushed garlic with extra virgin olive oil, Dijon, and lime juice. Drizzle over beans and serve.

Nutrition information per serving: Kcal: 197, Protein: 3.1g, Carbs: 11.7g, Fats: 17.2g

23. Chocolate Cocoa Balls

Ingredients:

½ cup of almond butter

1 cup of coconut, shredded

2 tablespoons of chia seeds

½ cup of cocoa powder, raw

½ cup of dark chocolate, shredded

¼ cup of almond milk

Preparation:

Combine the ingredients in a bowl and mix well to combine. Shape the balls using your hands and refrigerate for about 30 minutes.

Nutrition information per serving: Kcal: 259, Protein: 14.5g, Carbs: 65.9g, Fats: 38.6g

24.   Mushroom Sliders with Cauliflower Puree

Ingredients:

1 cup of fresh button mushrooms, chopped

3 tbsp of flax seeds

¾ cup of chia seeds

¾ cup of brown rice

¾ cup of buckwheat bread crumbs

1 tsp of tarragon

1 tsp of parsley, chopped

1 tsp of garlic powder

1 cup of fresh spinach, chopped

Preparation:

Pour 1 cup of water in a small saucepan. Bring it to a boil and cook rice until it's slightly sticky. This should take about 10 minutes.

At the same time, cook chia seeds until soft in a separate pot. Finely chop mushrooms. Thoroughly rinse spinach. Mix all the ingredients together in a large bowl. Put the bowl into the fridge to chill for 15 to 30 minutes.

Take mixture out of the fridge and form into patties. Make sure cooking surfaces are cleaned and greased before adding patties to prevent them from sticking. Fry each piece on a medium temperature for about 5 minutes on both sides.

Nutrition information per serving: Kcal: 490, Protein: 14.6g, Carbs: 89.3g, Fats: 7.5g

25.   Leafy Greens Smoothie

Ingredients:

¼ cup of roasted almonds, finely chopped

¼ cup of baby spinach, finely chopped

¼ cup of arugula, chopped

1 tbsp of almond butter

½ tsp of turmeric, ground

1 cup of rice milk

A handful of ice cubes

Preparation:

Toss all ingredients in a blender. Pulse to combine and transfer to a serving glasses. Serve immediately.

Nutrition information per serving: Kcal: 181, Protein: 4.6g, Carbs: 17.1g, Fats: 11.5g

26. Colorful Lentil Salad

Ingredients:

1 cup of lentils, pre-cooked

1 medium-sized spring onion, chopped

¼ cup of fresh parsley, chopped

½ tsp of salt

¼ tsp of black pepper, freshly ground

2 tbsp of olive oil

1 tbsp of sesame seeds

Preparation:

Palace the lentils in a deep pot and add 3 cups of water. Bring it to a boil and then reduce the heat to low. Cover with a lid and cook for 15 minutes more.

Remove from the heat and drain. Transfer to a bowl.

Now add all other ingredients, season with salt, pepper, olive oil, and sprinkle with sesame seeds. Toss well to combine.

Nutrition information per serving: Kcal: 981, Protein: 51.9g, Carbs: 119.8g, Fats: 34.7g

27.   Pumpkin Soup

Ingredients:

2 lb of pumpkin, pre-cooked

1 large onion, peeled and finely chopped

3 cups of vegetable broth

1 tbsp of turmeric, ground

½ cup of sour cream

½ tsp of salt

2 tbsp of fresh parsley

3 tbsp of olive oil

Preparation:

Place the pumpkin chops in a pot of boiling water. Cook until soften and remove from the heat. Set aside to cool and transfer to a food processor. Pulse until combined.

Now, combine onion, pureed pumpkin, turmeric, salt, and olive oil in a deep pot. Add vegetable broth and stir all well. Cover with a lid and cook for 1 hour on a low temperature. Add more water to adjust the thickness if needed. Remove from the heat and stir in the sour cream. Top with parsley and serve.

Nutrition information per serving: Kcal: 244, Protein: 3.8g, Carbs: 12.5g, Fats: 9.2g

28.   Baked Honey Apple Puree

Ingredients:

2 medium-sized apples, peeled and chopped

1 tbsp of fresh lime juice

2 tbsp of honey

½ tsp of cinnamon, ground

Preparation:

Preheat the oven to 375°F.

Wash and peel the apple. Combine the lemon juice with ground cinnamon and mix well. Spread this mixture over the apple using a kitchen brush.

Place the apple upright in a dish. Bake for about an hour, until the apple soften. Remove from the oven and let it cool for a while. Transfer to a food processor and blend until pureed. Transfer to a serving plate and top with honey.

Nutrition information per serving: Kcal: 181, Protein: 0.7g, Carbs: 48.6g, Fats: 0.4g

29.   Chocolate Buckwheat Muffins

Ingredients:

2 cups of buckwheat flour

3 tbsp of almond butter

1 cup of almond milk

4 tbsp of honey

1 tsp of baking powder

½ tsp of salt

2 tbsp of cocoa powder, raw

1 tsp of vanilla extract

1 tsp of lemon zest

Preparation:

Preheat oven to 325°F.

Line one 6-cup muffin tins with paper liners.

Combine all dry ingredients in a large bowl. Gently whisk in almond milk, almond butter, and beat well on high. Add water, lemon zest, and reduce the speed to low. Continue beating until well incorporated.

Using a spoon or ice cream scoop, divide the mixture evenly among the tins. Bake for 20-30 minutes, or until the toothpick inserted into the middle comes out clean. Remove from the oven and let it cool for a while. Serve with warm tea, honey, or a milk.

Nutrition information per serving: Kcal: 195, Protein: 4.8g, Carbs: 27.0g, Fats: 9.3g

30.   Green Goji Smoothie

Ingredients:

1 cup of baby spinach, finely chopped

½ medium-sized avocado, sliced

2 cups of water

1 cup of goji berries

1 tbsp of honey

1 tbsp of almond butter

Preparation:

Mix the ingredients in a blender and process for about 30 seconds.Transfer to a serving glasses and refrigerate for about 1 hour before serving.

Nutrition information per serving: Kcal: 193, Protein: 2.5g, Carbs: 28.9g, Fats: 8.6g

31.   Lentil Stew

Ingredients:

10 oz of lentils

3 tbsp of olive oil

1 medium-sized carrot, peeled and sliced

1 bay leaf

¼ cup of parsley, finely chopped

½ tbsp of turmeric, ground

½ tsp of salt

Preparation:

Preheat the oil in a medium skillet over a medium-high temperature. Add sliced carrot and parsley. Mix well and stir-fry for about 5 minutes.

Now add the lentils, bay leaf, some salt and turmeric. Add 4 cups of water and bring it to a boil. Reduce the heat, cover and cook until the lentils soften. This should take about an hour over a medium temperature. Stir occasionally.

Sprinkle with some parsley before serving.

Nutrition information per serving: Kcal: 702, Protein: 37.2g, Carbs: 89.7g, Fats: 22.7g

32.   Baby Spinach Salad with Apple Juice Dressing

Ingredients:

6 oz of baby spinach

½ cup of spring onions, chopped

3 tbsp of apple cider vinegar

¼ cup of fresh apple juice

2 tbsp of extra-virgin olive oil

1 tbsp of Dijon mustard

½ tsp of salt

Preparation:

Combine the apple juice with vinegar, olive oil, mustard, and salt. Mix well and set aside.

In a large bowl, combine baby spinach with chopped spring onions. Add apple dressing and mix well.

Serve.

Nutrition information per serving: Kcal: 172, Protein: 3.3g, Carbs: 9.1g, Fats: 14.7g

33. Detox Smoothie

Ingredients:

1 cup of coconut water

¼ cup of baby spinach, finely chopped

¼ cup of green tea

¼ cup of cucumber, peeled and chopped

¼ cup of avocado, chopped

1 tsp of vanilla extract

2 tsp of honey

Preparation:

Combine the ingredients in a blender. Blend for 40 seconds, or until nicely smooth. Serve immediately.

Nutrition information per serving: Kcal: 418, Protein: 3.8g, Carbs: 28.6g, Fats: 33.9g

34.　Braised Greens with Fresh Mint

Ingredients:

½ cup of brown rice

3 oz of fresh chicory, torn

3 oz wild asparagus, finely chopped

2 oz of fresh arugula, torn

3 oz of Swiss chard, torn

¼ cup of fresh mint, chopped

3 garlic cloves, crushed

¼ tsp of black pepper, freshly ground

1 tsp of salt

¼ cup of fresh lemon juice

3 tbsp of olive oil

Preparation:

Place rice in a pot. Add 1 ½ cups of water and bring it to a boil. Cook for about 10-12 minutes, or until the liquid evaporates. Stir occasionally. Remove from the heat and set aside.

Fill a large pot with salted water and add greens. Bring it to a boil and cook for 2-3 minutes. Remove from the heat and drain.

In a medium-sized skillet, heat up 3 tablespoons of olive oil. Add crushed garlic and stir-fry for about 2-3 minutes. Now add the greens, salt, pepper, and about half of the lemon juice. Stir-fry the greens for five more minutes. Add rice and mix well again.

Remove from the heat. Season with more lemon juice and serve.

Nutrition information per serving: Kcal: 269, Protein: 5.0g, Carbs: 30.1g, Fats: 15.4g

35. Hummus

Ingredients:

14 oz of chickpeas, pre-cooked

2 tbsp of lemon juice

2 tbsp of olive oil

2 cloves garlic, crushed

1 tbsp of parsley, finely chopped

3 tbsp tahini

Preparation:

Place chickpeas in a pot of boiling water and cook until soften. Remove from the heat and drain well. Let it cool for a while.

Combine the ingredients in a food processor and blend until pureed. Serve immediately or keep it refrigerated in a jar.

Nutrition information per serving: Kcal: 328, Protein: 14.2g, Carbs: 42.2g, Fats: 12.8g

36.   Rice Yogurt with Fresh Plums and Chia Seeds

Ingredients:

2 tbsp of chia seeds

½ cup of almond milk

½ cup of Greek yogurt

2 oz of white quinoa

½ cup of water

2 medium-sized plums, pitted and sliced

1 tbsp of honey

Preparation:

Combine the water and almond milk in a medium sized saucepan. Bring it to a boil and add quinoa. Reduce the heat and cook for about 20 minutes, or until all the liquid evaporates.

Transfer the cooked quinoa to a bowl. Stir in the rice yogurt, honey, and chia seeds.

Top with sliced plums and serve.

Nutrition information per serving: Kcal: 223, Protein: 6.6g, Carbs: 26.5g, Fats: 11.4g

37.   Creamy Pea Puree

Ingredients:

1 cup of green peas, pre-cooked

1 tbsp of olive oil

1 small onion, finely chopped

1 cup of skim milk

2 tbsp of tahini

½ cup of spinach, chopped

1 garlic clove, crushed

½ tsp of salt

Preparation:

Place peas in a pot of boiling water. Sprinkle with some salt and cook for 30 minutes, or until soften. Remove from the heat and set aside to cool.

Combine the ingredients in a food processor and beat to combine. Transfer to a dish with a lid or a jar. Keep in the refrigerator for 2-3 days.

Nutrition information per serving: Kcal: 135, Protein: 5.6g, Carbs: 11.9g, Fats: 7.7g

38.   Creamy Broccoli and Rice Casserole

Ingredients:

2 cups of broccoli, chopped

7 oz Brussels sprouts, halved

1 cup of quinoa, rinsed

4 cups of vegetable broth

2 small onions, finely chopped

1 cup of cashew cream, homemade

2 tsp dry thyme, crushed

4 tbsp of extra-virgin olive oil

¼ tsp of salt

¼ tsp of black pepper, ground

Preparation:

Preheat the oven to 400°F.

Combine quinoa, vegetable broth, and dry thyme in a large saucepan. Add some salt and pepper to taste and bring it to a boil. Reduce the heat and cook until the liquid is absorbed, about 12-15 minutes. Remove from the heat and set aside.

Preheat the oil in a large nonstick saucepan over a medium-high temperature. Add onions and stir-fry for about 2-3 minutes, or until translucent. Now, add chopped broccoli and Brussel sprouts. Continue to cook for 10 more minutes, or until vegetable tender-crisp.

Combine the broccoli mixture with quinoa in a large bowl. Add cashew cream and stir well. Place in a lightly oiled shallow casserole dish. Bake for about 20 minutes, or until the top is lightly charred and crisp.

For the homemade cashew cream, soak the cashews in filtered water for about an hour. Drain and transfer to a powerful food processor. Add juice of one lemon and 1 teaspoon of kosher salt. Mix well until smooth.

Nutrition information per serving: Kcal: 282, Protein: 9.8g, Carbs: 25.3g, Fats: 17.1g

39. Button Mushrooms Soup

Ingredients:

1lb of fresh button mushrooms, finely sliced

2 garlic cloves, crushed

1 medium-sized onion, finely chopped

5 cups vegetable broth

4 tbsp extra-virgin olive oil

½ tsp of sea salt

1 tbsp of fresh parsley, finely chopped

¼ cup of fresh thyme, finely chopped

Preparation:

Preheat the oil in a large saucepan over a medium-high temperature. Add onion and garlic, and stir-fry for 2-3 minutes, or until translucent.

Now, add mushrooms, thyme, salt, and vegetable broth. Bring it to a boil and then reduce the heat to low. Cover with a lid and cook for about 7-10 minutes, or until mushrooms soften. Remove from the heat and serve immediately.

Sprinkle with some fresh parsley before serving.

Nutrition information per serving: Kcal: 143, Protein: 6.9g, Carbs: 6.6g, Fats: 10.9g

40.   Strawberries Almond Cream

Ingredients:

1 cup of almond yogurt

1 cup of strawberries, chopped

½ cup of almonds, minced

1 tbsp of honey

1 tsp of cocoa, raw

Preparation:

Combine almond yogurt and strawberries in a medium bowl. Using a hand mixer, blend on a low speed for 1 minutes. Stir in the almonds with a spoon and transfer to a serving bowls. Top with honey and cocoa and serve imediatelly.

Nutrition information per serving: Kcal: 470, Protein: 8.4g, Carbs: 26.4g, Fats: 40.8g

41.   Red Lentil Soup

Ingredients:

1 cup of red lentils, soaked

1 medium-sized onion, finely chopped

2 large carrots, chopped

½ cup of sour cream

1 tbsp of all-purpose flour

½ tsp of black pepper, ground

½ tsp of cumin, ground

½ tsp of salt

2 tbsp of olive oil

Preparation:

Place the carrots and sour cream in a food processor and blend until smooth. Set aside.

Preheat the oil in a deep pot over a medium-high temperature. Add onion and stir-fry for 5 minutes, or until translucent. Add the flour and cook for 10 more minutes, stirring constantly.

Add carrot puree, red lentils, and sprinkle with pepper, cumin, and salt. Pour about 4 cups of water and stir well. Bring it to a boil and then reduce the heat to low. Cover with a lid and cook for 1 hour. Add more water to adjust the thickness if needed while cooking.

Remove from the heat and serve warm.

Nutrition information per serving: Kcal: 201, Protein: 18.9g, Carbs: 50.6g, Fats: 18.2g

42. Sweet Potato with Red Cabbage & Carrots Cream

Ingredients:

1 medium-sized sweet potato, peeled and chopped

2 cups of red cabbage

2 large spring onions, sliced

2 medium-sized carrots, sliced

¼ cup of extra-virgin olive oil

2 tbsp of fresh lemon juice

½ tsp of sea salt

½ tsp of black pepper, freshly ground

Preparation:

Place sweet potato in a pot of a boiling water. Cook until soften and remove from the heat. Cut the potato into bite-sized pieces and transfer to a large bowl. Set aside.

Combine olive oil, lemon juice, salt, and pepper. Mix well and set aside.

Place cabbage chops and carrots in a food processor. Pulse quickly until chopped roughly. Transfer the mixture to a bowl with potatoes and stir well to combine. Sprinkle with dressing and mix all again.

Serve immediately.

Nutrition information per serving: Kcal: 215, Protein: 2.1g, Carbs: 16.2g, Fats: 17.0g

43.   Mint Veggie Smoothie

Ingredients:

2 cups of baby spinach, roughly chopped

1 cup of almond milk

½ cup of avocado, peeled and chopped

½ cup fresh mint leaves

½ cup of water

1 tbsp of honey

¼ cup of coconut milk

Preparation:

Combine all ingredients in a food processor and pulse until nicely smooth. Serve immediately.

Nutrition information per serving: Kcal: 312, Protein: 3.8g, Carbs: 15.4g, Fats: 28.8g

44.   Kidney Bean Salad

Ingredients:

9 oz of kidney beans, pre-cooked

1 medium-sized cucumber, sliced

½ cup of spring onions, chopped

1 cup of radishes, sliced

1 tbsp of fresh celery, chopped

For the marinade:

¼ cup of olive oil

3 tbsp of apple cider vinegar

1 tsp of fresh thyme, finely chopped

½ tsp of salt

¼ tsp of black pepper, ground

Preparation:

Place the beans in a pot of boiling water and cook until soften. Remove from the heat and drain well. Set aside to cool for a while.

Combine all marinade ingredients in a bowl. Mix well and

chill for about 15 minutes in the refrigerator to allow flavors to meld.

Meanwhile, combine the beans with vegetables in a bowl. Drizzle with some marinade and serve.

Nutrition information per serving: Kcal: 347, Protein: 15.3g, Carbs: 44.1g, Fats: 13.4g

45. Fresh Kiwi Smoothie

Ingredients:

1 cup of coconut milk

3 medium-sized kiwis, peeled and sliced

1 medium-sized banana

1 tsp of ginger, freshly grated

2 tbsp of chia seeds

Preparation:

Place the ingredients in a food processor and pulse to combine. Transfer the mixture to a serving glasses and serve immediately.

Nutrition information per serving: Kcal: 221, Protein: 7.4g, Carbs: 37.3g, Fats: 27.3g

46.   Easy White Chili

Ingredients:

2 cups of white beans, pre-cooked

2 tbsp of all-purpose flour

2 tbsp of olive oil

1 small onion, chopped

1 tbsp of fresh parsley, finely chopped

1 tsp of chili pepper, ground

¼ tsp of salt

Preparation:

Place the beans in a deep pot. Add enough water to cover and cook for about 2-3 minutes. Remove from the heat, drain and rinse. Wash the pot and pour fresh water in it. Add boiled beans and cook again for about 45 minutes, or until beans soften. Drain and set aside.

Heat up the olive oil in a large nonstick saucepan over a medium-high temperature. Add chopped onion and stir-fry until translucent. Stir in the flour and cook for 1 minute.

Now, add beans, parsley, chili pepper, and salt.Add enough

water to cover all ingredients and reduce the heat to low. Cook for about 1 hour.

You can reduce the cooking time with a pressure cooker. Set the heat to high, securely lock the lid and cook for 20 minutes.

Nutrition information per serving: Kcal: 558, Protein: 32.3g, Carbs: 87.6g, Fats: 10.6g

47. Cauliflower Puree

Ingredients:

8 oz of cauliflower, chopped

1 cup of fresh spinach, chopped

½ tsp of sea salt

¼ tsp of black pepper, ground

1 tsp of dry mint, minced

¼ tsp of red pepper flakes

Water

Preparation:

Wash and roughly chop the cauliflower. Cook for about 15-20 minutes in salted water. When done, drain and mash it with a fork. Add dry mint and some more salt. If the mixture is too thick, you can add some more water. Sprinkle with red pepper flakes and serve

Nutrition information per serving: Kcal: 232, Protein: 4.6g, Carbs: 12.5g, Fats: 0.3g

48.   Rice Noodles with Sweet Cashew Pasta

Ingredients:

14 oz of rice noodles

2 tbsp of olive oil

2 tsp of turmeric, ground

2 cups of coconut milk

½ cup of sour cashew cream

2 tbsp of almond butter

¼ cup of fresh lime juice

¼ cup of toasted cashews

1 tsp of honey, raw

1 medium-sized onion, finely chopped

1 tbsp of fresh ginger, grated

¼ tsp of salt

Preparation:

Soak the noodles for 5 minutes. Drain and set aside.

Preheat the oil in a large saucepan over a medium-high

temperature. Add turmeric and briefly, cook for about a minute. Now, add coconut milk and bring it to a boil. Reduce the heat and add almond butter, cashew cream, fresh lime juice, cashews, onion, and fresh ginger. Continue to cook for about 5 minutes.

Add noodles and honey. Sprinkle with some salt and mix well. Cover and allow it to warm up. Serve.

Nutrition information per serving: Kcal: 446, Protein: 6.6g, Carbs: 32.1g, Fats: 35.0g

49.   Creamy Leblebi Soup

Ingredients:

7 oz of chickpeas, soaked overnight

1 large tomato, peeled and finely chopped

1 medium-sized red onion, finely chopped

1 tbsp of cumin, ground

2 cups of vegetable broth

2 tbsp of olive oil

2 tbsp of butter

1 tbsp of Cayenne pepper

1 tsp of salt

2 tbsp of fresh parsley, finely chopped

Preparation:

Grease the bottom of a deep pot with olive oil and place roughly chopped tomato and onion. Stir-fry for 3 minutes over a medium-high temperature. Now, add cumin, chickpeas, and vegetable broth. Bring it to a boil, and then reduce the heat to low. Cover with a lid and cook for 3 hours. Remove from the heat and set aside to cool.

Transfer the mixture to a food processor. Stir in the butter and Cayenne pepper. Pulse until well incorporated. Return the mixture to the pot and add water to adjust the thickness, if needed. Heat up the soup and season with salt and chopped parsley before serving.

Nutrition information per serving: Kcal: 340, Protein: 13.2g, Carbs: 36.3g, Fats: 17.1g

50. Hot Mexican Wraps

Ingredients:

3 large lettuce leaves

½ cup of red beans, cooked

½ cup of green beans, chopped

½ cup of fresh arugula, chopped

½ small red onion, finely chopped

¼ tsp of Himalayan salt

1 tsp of apple cider vinegar

Preparation:

Combine red and green beans in a pot of boiling water. Cook until soften and remove from the heat. Drain well and set aside.

In a large bowl, combine red beans, green beans, onion, and arugula. Season with apple cider vinegar and some salt to taste.

Place 2 tablespoons of this mixture over each lettuce leaf. Wrap and secure with a toothpick. Sprinkle with lemon juice and serve.

Nutrition information per serving: Kcal: 345, Protein: 22.4g, Carbs: 64.0g, Fats: 1.2g

JUICE RECIPES

1.   Mango Lemon Juice

Ingredients:

1 cup mango, cubed

1 large lemon, peeled

1 cup sweet cherries, pitted

1 cup watermelon, cubed

1 tbsp liquid honey

2 oz water

Preparation:

Peel the mango and cut into small chunks. Set aside.

Peel the lemon and cut lengthwise in half. Set aside.

Wash the cherries under cold running water. Drain and cut in half. Remove the pits and set aside.

Cut the watermelon lengthwise. For one cup, you will need about 1 large wedge. Peel and cut into chunks. Remove the seeds and set aside. Reserve the rest of the melon for some other juices.

Now, process mango, lemon, cherries, and watermelon in a juicer.

Transfer to serving glasses and add few ice cubes before serving.

Enjoy!

Nutrition information per serving: Kcal: 288, Protein: 4.6g, Carbs: 68.3g, Fats: 1.3g

2.   Carrot Melon Juice

Ingredients:

1 large carrot, sliced

1 large wedge of honeydew melon, peeled and cubed

1 cup cucumber, sliced

1 small ginger knob, 1-inch thick

1/8 tsp turmeric powder

2 oz water

Preparation:

Wash and peel the carrot. Cut into thin slices and set aside.

Cut melon lengthwise in half. Scoop out the seeds and then wash. Cut one large wedge and peel it. Cut into small cubes and set aside.

Wash the cucumber and cut into thin slices. Fill the measuring cup and reserve the rest for later. Set aside.

Peel the ginger knob and cut into small pieces. Set aside.

Now, combine carrot, melon, and cucumber in a juicer and process until juiced. Transfer to a serving glass and stir in the turmeric and water.

Refrigerate for 5 minutes before serving.

Nutrition information per serving: Kcal: 92, Protein: 2.6g, Carbs: 25.7g, Fats: 0.5g

3.   Agave Blueberry Juice

Ingredients:

2 cups fresh blueberries

1 cup black grapes

1 cup fresh mint, torn

1 large banana, peeled

1 tsp agave nectar

Preparation:

Place the blueberries in a colander. Rinse well under cold running water and drain. Set aside.

Wash the grapes and remove the stems. Fill the measuring cup and reserve the rest in the refrigerator. Set aside.

Wash the mint thoroughly under cold running water. Drain and torn into small pieces. Set aside.

Now, combine blueberries, grapes, mint, and banana in a juicer and process until juiced. Transfer to a serving glass and stir in the agave nectar.

Refrigerate for 5 minutes before serving.

Nutrition information per serving: Kcal: 326, Protein: 6.2g, Carbs: 93.4g, Fats: 2.1g

4.   Strawberry Ginger Juice

Ingredients:

1 cup fresh strawberries, chopped

1 small ginger knob, 1-inch thick

1 cup fresh kale, torn

1 whole lemon, peeled

Preparation:

Wash the strawberries under cold running water. Drain and set aside.

Peel the ginger knob and finely chop into tiny pieces. Set aside.

Place the kale in a colander and rinse thoroughly under cold running water. Drain and torn into small pieces. Set aside.

Peel the lemon and cut lengthwise in half. Set aside.

Combine strawberries, ginger, kale, and lemon in a juicer and process until juiced.

Transfer to serving glasses add some ice cubes before serving.

Enjoy!

Nutritional information per serving: Kcal: 120, Protein: 5.9g, Carbs: 38.6g, Fats: 1.8g

5. Beet Apple Juice

Ingredients:

1 cup beet greens

1 medium-sized Granny Smith's apple, chopped

1 cup cantaloupe, diced

1 tbsp fresh mint, chopped

1 cup cauliflower, chopped

Preparation:

Wash the beet greens and torn with hands. Set aside.

Wash the apple and cut lengthwise in half. Remove the core and cut into bite-sized pieces. Set aside.

Cut the cantaloupe in half. Scoop out the seeds and flesh. Cut two wedges and peel them. Chop into chunks and set aside. Reserve the rest of the cantaloupe in a refrigerator.

Trim off the outer leaves of cauliflower. Wash it and cut into small pieces. Reserve the rest in the refrigerator.

Soak the mint leaves in hot water. Let it stand for 2 minutes.

Now, process beet greens, apple, cantaloupe, cauliflower,

and mint in a juicer.

Transfer to serving glasses and stir in the mint soaking water.

Refrigerate for 10-15 minutes before serving and enjoy.

Nutritional information per serving: Kcal: 123, Protein: 8.1g, Carbs: 37.7g, Fats: 1.1g

6.   Grapefruit Orange Juice

Ingredients:

1 whole grapefruit, peeled

1 large orange, peeled

1 cup pineapple, chunked

1 cup cauliflower, chopped

¼ cup pure coconut water, unsweetened

Preparation:

Peel the grapefruit and orange and divide into wedges. Set aside.

Cut the top of a pineapple and peel it using a sharp knife. Cut into small chunks. Reserve the rest of the pineapple in a refrigerator.

Trim off the outer leaves of cauliflower. Wash it and cut into small pieces. Reserve the rest in the refrigerator.

Now, combine grapefruit, orange, pineapple, and cauliflower in a juicer and process until juiced. Transfer to serving glasses and stir in the pure coconut water.

Add few ice cubes and serve immediately.

Nutritional information per serving: Kcal: 247, Protein: 6.5g, Carbs: 74g, Fats: 1g

7.   Squash Nutmeg Juice

Ingredients:

1 cup butternut squash, chunked

1 cup avocado, chunked

½ tsp cinnamon, freshly ground

¼ tsp nutmeg, ground

¼ cup water

Preparation:

Peel the squash and cut in half. Scoop out the seeds using a spoon. Cut about 2 large wedges and pee. Cut the wedges into small chunks and fill the measuring cup. Reserve the rest in the refrigerator.

Peel and cut the avocado in half. Remove the pit and cut into small chunks. Set aside.

Now, combine squash and avocado in a juicer and process until juiced.

Transfer to serving glasses and stir in the water and cinnamon.

Serve immediately.

Nutritional information per serving: Kcal: 256, Protein: 5.3g, Carbs: 27.8g, Fats: 22.3g

8. Blackberry Mint Juice

Ingredients:

1 cup blackberries

1 cup fresh mint, torn

1 cup cantaloupe, chopped

1 large orange, peeled

¼ tsp cinnamon, ground

Preparation:

Place the blackberries in a colander and rinse well. Drain and set aside.

Rinse the mint under cold running water and drain. Torn into small pieces and set aside.

Cut the cantaloupe in half. Scrape out the seeds and cut one large wedge. Peel and chop into small pieces. Fill the measuring cup and wrap the rest in a plastic foil. Refrigerate for later.

Peel the orange and divide into wedges. Cut each wedge in half and set aside.

Now, combine blackberries, mint, cantaloupe, and orange

in a juicer and process until juiced. Transfer to a serving glass and stir in the cinnamon. Optionally, add some water to increase the juice amount.

Serve immediately.

Nutrition information per serving: Kcal: 157, Protein: 5.9g, Carbs: 51.9g, Fats: 1.5g

9. Cinnamon Pineapple Juice

Ingredients:

1 cup pineapple, chunked

1 whole lime, peeled and halved

1 small Granny Smith's apple, peeled and cored

1 tsp fresh mint leaves, finely chopped

¼ tsp cinnamon, ground

Preparation:

Cut the top of a pineapple and peel it using a sharp knife. Cut into small chunks and fill the measuring cup. Reserve the rest in the refrigerator.

Peel the lime and cut lengthwise in half. Set aside.

Wash the apple and remove the core. Cut into bite-sized pieces and set aside.

Process pineapple, lime, and apple in a juicer. Transfer to serving glasses and stir in the cinnamon. Add more water if needed.

Garnish with mint leaves and refrigerate before serving.

Nutritional information per serving: Kcal: 153, Protein: 1.7g, Carbs: 46.7g, Fats: 0.6g

10.   Mango Ginger Juice

Ingredients:

1 cup mango, chunked

1 small ginger slice

1 cup pomegranate seeds

1 medium-sized Gala apple, cored

1 oz coconut water

Preparation:

Peel the mango and cut into chunks. Fill the measuring cup and reserve the rest in the refrigerator. Set aside.

Peel the ginger slice and chop into small pieces. Set aside.

Cut the top of the pomegranate fruit using a sharp paring knife. Slice down to each of the white membranes inside of the fruit. Pop the seeds into a measuring cup and set aside.

Wash the apple and cut lengthwise in half. Remove the core and cut into small pieces. Set aside.

Now, combine mango, ginger, pomegranate seeds, and apple in a juicer and process until juiced. Transfer to a serving glass and stir in the cinnamon and water.

Refrigerate for 5 minutes before serving.

Nutrition information per serving: Kcal: 227, Protein: 3.6g, Carbs: 64.1g, Fats: 1.9g

11. Orange Honey Juice

Ingredients:

3 large red oranges, peeled

1 tbsp honey, raw

1 large banana, peeled

1 tbsp fresh mint leaves, finely chopped

Preparation:

Peel the oranges and divide into wedges. Set aside.

Peel the banana and cut into small chunks. Set aside.

Process banana and oranges in a juicer. Transfer to serving glasses and stir in the honey.

Garnish with mint and refrigerate for 10 minutes before serving.

Enjoy!

Nutritional information per serving: Kcal: 123, Protein: 4.1g, Carbs: 73.9g, Fats: 1.1g

12. Mint Cucumber Juice

Ingredients:

1 large honeydew melon wedge, chopped

1 cup fresh mint, chopped

1 medium-sized cucumber, chopped

1 small Golden delicious apple, cored

1 oz coconut water

Preparation:

Place mint in a colander and wash thoroughly. Slightly drain and chop into small pieces. Set aside.

Wash the cucumber and cut into thin slices. Set aside.

Cut the melon in half. Cut one large wedge and peel the peel it. Cut into small pieces and set aside. Wrap the rest of the melon in a plastic foil and refrigerate for later.

Wash the apple and cut lengthwise in half. Remove the core and cut into bite-sized pieces. Set aside.

Now, combine mint, cucumber, melon, and apple in a juicer and process until juiced.

Transfer to a serving glass and stir in the water. Optionally, add 1 tablespoon of lemon juice for a better taste. Refrigerate for 10 minutes before serving.

Enjoy!

Nutrition information per serving: Kcal: 139, Protein: 4.1g, Carbs: 40.5g, Fats: 0.9g

13.   Sour Cherry Juice

Ingredients:

2 cups sour cherries, pitted

1 medium-sized watermelon slice

1 cup celery, chopped

1 small ginger knob, peeled

1 oz water

Preparation:

Cut the watermelon in half. Cut one medium-sized wedge and wrap the rest in a plastic foil and refrigerate. Dice the wedge and remove the pits. Set aside.

Wash the celery and cut into small pieces. Fill the measuring cup and reserve the rest for later. Set aside.

Rinse the cherries under cold running water using a colander. Drain and cut each in half. Remove the pits and set aside.

Peel the ginger knob and cut into small pieces. Set aside.

Now, combine cherries, watermelon, celery, and ginger knob in a juicer and process until juiced. Transfer to a serving glass and stir in the water. Optionally, you can use coconut water if you like.

Serve immediately.

Nutrition information per serving: Kcal: 143, Protein: 3.4g, Carbs: 40.2g, Fats: 0.7g

14.   Sweet Berry Juice

Ingredients:

1 cup fresh cranberries

1 cup fresh blueberries

3 small Granny Smith's apples, cored

1 cup fresh kale, torn

1 tbsp liquid honey

Preparation:

Combine cranberries and blueberries in a colander and wash under cold running water. Drain and set aside.

Wash the apples and remove the core. Cut into bite-sized pieces and set aside.

Wash the kale thoroughly and torn with hands. Set aside.

Now, process cranberries, blueberries, apples, and kale in a juicer.

Transfer to serving glasses and stir in the honey. Add some ice or refrigerate before serving.

Nutrition information per serving: Kcal: 368, Protein: 5.6g, Carbs: 106g, Fats: 2.2g

15.   Cabbage Ginger Juice

Ingredients:

1 cup purple cabbage, chopped

1 small ginger knob, peeled and chopped

1 cup cauliflower, chopped

1 cup carrots, sliced

1 cup collard greens, chopped

Preparation:

Combine cabbage and collard greens in a colander. Wash thoroughly under cold running water and slightly drain. Chop into small pieces and set aside.

Peel the ginger knob and finely chop. Set aside.

Wash the cauliflower and trim off the outer leaves. Cut into bite-sized pieces and fill the measuring cup. Reserve the rest for later.

Wash and peel the carrots. Cut into thin slices and fill the measuring cup. Set aside.

Now, combine cabbage, ginger, cauliflower, carrots, and collard greens in a juicer and process until juiced. Transfer to a serving glass and refrigerate for 10 minutes before serving.

Nutrition information per serving: Kcal: 138, Protein: 5.3g, Carbs: 40.3g, Fats: 0.8g

16.   Apple Carrot Juice

Ingredients:

2 large Gala apples, peeled and cored

3 medium-sized carrots, sliced

1 cup parsnips, sliced

¼ cup water

1 tbsp fresh lemon juice

Preparation:

Wash the apples and remove the core. Cut into bite-sized pieces and set aside.

Wash the carrots and parsnips and cut into thick slices. Set aside.

Now, combine apples, carrots, and parsnips in a juicer and process until juiced.

Transfer to serving glasses and stir in the water and lemon juice. Garnish with some mint and refrigerate before serving.

Enjoy!

Nutritional information per serving: Kcal: 332, Protein: 5.4g, Carbs: 100g, Fats: 1.6g

17.   Melon Blueberry Juice

Ingredients:

1 large wedge of honeydew melon

1 cup fresh blueberries

1 whole lemon, peeled and halved

1 large cucumber, sliced

Preparation:

Cut the honeydew melon lengthwise in half. Scoop out the seeds using a spoon. Cut the large wedges and peel them. Cut into small chunks and place in a bowl. Wrap the rest of the melon in a plastic foil and refrigerate.

Rinse the blueberries under cold running water. Drain and set aside.

Peel the lemon and cut lengthwise in half. Set aside.

Wash the cucumber and cut into thin slices. Set aside.

Now, process honeydew melon, blueberries, lemon, and cucumber in a juicer.

Transfer to serving glasses and add some ice if you like.

Serve immediately.

Nutritional information per serving: Kcal: 202, Protein: 5.5g, Carbs: 59.3g, Fats: 1.7g

18.   Green Tomato Juice

Ingredients:

2 cups Iceberg lettuce, chopped

1 cup mustard greens, torn

1 cup parsley, torn

1 whole cucumber, sliced

1 large tomato, chopped

¼ tsp salt

Preparation:

Rinse the lettuce thoroughly under cold running water. Chop into small pieces and set aside.

Combine mustard greens and parsley in a large colander. Rinse well and drain. Torn into small pieces and set aside.

Wash the cucumber and cut into thin slices. Set aside.

Wash the tomato and place in a bowl. Chop into bite-sized pieces and reserve the tomato juice while cutting. Set aside.

Now, combine lettuce, mustard greens, parsley, cucumber, and tomato in a juicer and process until juiced. Transfer to a serving glass and stir in the turmeric, salt, and reserved tomato juice.

Refrigerate for 5 minutes before serving.

Enjoy!

Nutrition information per serving: Kcal: 85, Protein: 7.6g, Carbs: 25.3g, Fats: 1.6g

19.   Sweet Orange Juice

Ingredients:

1 large orange, peeled

1 large peach, peeled

1 cup parsnip, sliced

1 tsp agave nectar

Preparation:

Wash the peach and cut in half. Remove the pit and cut into bite-sized pieces. Set aside.

Wash the parsnips and cut into thick slices. Set aside.

Peel the orange and divide into wedges. Set aside.

Now, process orange, peach, and parsnip in a juicer. Transfer to serving glasses and stir in the agave syrup.

Add some ice and serve immediately.

Nutritional information per serving: Kcal: 177, Protein: 5.2g, Carbs: 53.7g, Fats: 1.1g

20.   Carrot Kiwi Juice

Ingredients:

2 whole kiwis, peeled

1 cup carrots, chopped

2 cups green cabbage, shredded

1 whole grapefruit, peeled

1 tbsp honey, raw

Preparation:

Wash the carrots and cut into small pieces. Set aside.

Peel the kiwis and cut in half. Set aside.

Wash the cabbage thoroughly and roughly chop it using hands. Set aside.

Wash the grapefruit and cut into chunks. Set aside.

Now, process carrots, kiwis, cabbage, and grapefruit in a juicer. Transfer to a serving glass and stir in the honey.

Serve immediately.

Nutritional information per serving: Kcal: 219, Protein: 6.9g, Carbs: 69g, Fats: 1.5g

21.   Apple Cantaloupe Juice

Ingredients:

1 small Red Delicious apple, cored

1 cup cantaloupe, cubed

1 cup fresh kale, torn

1 cup beets, sliced

¼ tsp ginger, ground

Preparation:

Wash the apple and cut lengthwise in half. Remove the core and cut into bite-sized pieces. Set aside.

Cut the cantaloupe in half. Scrape out the seeds and cut one large wedge. Peel and chop into small pieces. Fill the measuring cup and wrap the rest in a plastic foil. Refrigerate for later.

Rinse the kale thoroughly under cold running water. Drain and torn into small pieces. Set aside.

Wash the beets and trim off the green ends. Cut into thin slices and fill the measuring cup. Reserve the rest for some other juice.

Now, combine apple, cantaloupe, kale, and beets in a juicer and process until juiced. Transfer to a serving glass and stir in the ginger.

Add some ice and serve immediately.

Nutrition information per serving: Kcal: 181, Protein: 7g, Carbs: 51.1g, Fats: 1.4g

22.　Sweet Cucumber Melon Juice

Ingredients:

1 large cucumber, sliced

1 large honeydew melon wedge, chopped

1 cup watermelon, seeded

1 cup cantaloupe, cubed

1 tbsp liquid honey

Preparation:

Wash the cucumber and cut into thick slices. Set aside.

Cut the honeydew melon lengthwise in half. Scoop out the seeds using a spoon. Cut one large wedge and peel. Cut into small chunks and place in a bowl. Wrap the rest of the melon in a plastic foil and refrigerate.

Cut the watermelon lengthwise. For one cup, you will need about 1 large wedge. Peel and cut into chunks. Remove the seeds and set aside. Reserve the rest of for some other juices.

Cut the cantaloupe in half. Scoop out the seeds and flesh. Cut two wedges and peel them. Chop into chunks and set aside. Reserve the rest of the cantaloupe in a refrigerator.

Now, process cucumber, honeydew melon, watermelon, and cantaloupe in a juicer.

Transfer to serving glasses and stir in the honey.

Serve immediately and enjoy!

Nutritional information per serving: Kcal: 201, Protein: 3.4g, Carbs: 57.6g, Fats: 0.8g

23.   Guava Lime Juice

Ingredients:

1 large guava, peeled

1 large lime, peeled

1 large cucumber

1 ripe avocado, pitted and peeled

2 oz coconut water

Preparation:

Peel the guava and cut into small chunks. Set aside.

Peel the lime and cut lengthwise in half. Set aside.

Wash the cucumber and cut into thick slices. Set aside.

Peel the avocado and cut in half. Remove the pit and cut into chunks. Set aside.

Now, process guava, lime, cucumber, and avocado in a juicer. Transfer to serving glasses and stir in the coconut water. Optionally, add some ginger if you like a bitter taste.

Add some ice and serve immediately.

Nutrition information per serving: Kcal: 352, Protein: 7.6g, Carbs: 41.6g, Fats: 30.3g

24.   Carrot Apple Juice

Ingredients:

1 large carrot, sliced

1 small Granny Smith's apple, cored and chopped

1 cup mango, chunked

1 medium-sized orange, wedged

1 oz coconut water

Preparation:

Wash and peel the carrot. Cut into bite-sized pieces and set aside.

Wash the apple and cut in half. Remove the core and cut into bite-sized pieces. Set aside.

Peel the mango and cut into chunks. Fill the measuring cup and reserve the rest for later.

Peel the orange and divide into wedges. Set aside.

Now, combine carrot, apple, mango, and orange in a juicer and process until juiced. Transfer to a serving glass and stir in the coconut water.

Serve immediately and enjoy!

Nutrition information per serving: Kcal: 189, Protein: 2.6g, Carbs: 56.4g, Fats:1.1g

25.   Sweet Coconut Juice

Ingredients:

½ cup pure coconut water, unsweetened

1 tsp agave nectar

1 Red Delicious apple, peeled and cored

1 medium-sized artichoke, chopped

1 cup fresh spinach, torn

½ tsp ginger, freshly ground

Preparation:

Wash the apple and remove the core. Cut into bite-sized pieces and set aside.

Using a sharp knife, trim off the outer leave of the artichoke. Cut into small pieces and set aside.

Rinse the spinach thoroughly under cold running water. Drain and torn into small pieces. Set aside.

Now, process apple, artichoke, and spinach in a juicer.

Transfer to serving glasses and stir in the ginger, coconut water, and agave nectar.

Add some ice and serve immediately.

Nutritional information per serving: Kcal: 195, Protein: 13.7g, Carbs: 63.4g, Fats: 1.3g

26.   Guava Lemon Juice

Ingredients:

1 whole guava, chopped

2 whole lemons, peeled

1 cup pineapple chunks

2 cups spinach, chopped

½ cup coconut water, unsweetened

Preparation:

Wash the guava and cut into chunks. If you are using large fruit, reserve the rest for some other recipe in a refrigerator.

Peel the lemons and cut lengthwise in half. Set aside.

Cut the top of a pineapple and peel it using a sharp knife. Cut into small chunks. Reserve the rest in the refrigerator.

Rinse the spinach thoroughly under cold running water. Torn with your hands and set aside.

Now, process guava, lemons, pineapple, and spinach and in a juicer. Transfer to serving glasses and stir in the coconut water.

Add some ice and serve immediately.

Nutritional information per serving: Kcal: 130, Protein: 4.8g, Carbs: 43g, Fats: 1.2g

27.   Beet Cauliflower Juice

Ingredients:

1 cup beets, trimmed

1 cup beet greens, chopped

1 cup cauliflower, chopped

1 cup parsnips, chopped

2 tbsp fresh mint, chopped

Preparation:

Wash the beets and trim off the green parts. Cut into small pieces. Chop the greens and set aside.

Trim off the outer leaves of a cauliflower. Wash it and chop into small pieces. Set aside.

Rinse the parsnips and cut into thick slices. Set aside.

Now, process beets, beet greens, cauliflower, and parsnips in a juicer.Transfer to serving glasses and garnish with some fresh mint before serving.

Enjoy!

Nutritional information per serving: Kcal: 166, Protein: 9.9g, Carbs: 52.3g, Fats: 1.5g

28.   Pineapple Mint Juice

Ingredients:

1 cup pineapple, chunked

1 cup fresh mint, torn

1 cup cucumber, sliced

1 whole guava, chopped

1 oz coconut water

Preparation:

Cut the top of the pineapple and peel it using a sharp paring knife. Peel it and cut into small pieces. Fill the measuring cup and reserve the rest in the refrigerator. Set aside.

Wash the mint and slightly drain. Torn with hands and set aside.

Wash the cucumber and cut into thin slices. Fill the measuring cup and reserve the rest in the refrigerator.

Wash and peel the guava fruit. Chop into bite-sized pieces and set aside.

Now, combine pineapple, mint, cucumber, and guava in a juicer and process until juiced. Transfer to a serving glass and stir in the water.

Refrigerate for 5 minutes before serving.

Nutrition information per serving: Kcal: 115, Protein: 3.6g, Carbs: 35.2g, Fats: 1.1g

29. Avocado Lime Juice

Ingredients:

1 cup avocado, peeled and pitted

1 large lime, peeled

2 large honeydew melon wedges

5 tbsp fresh mint

1 medium-sized pineapple slice, chopped

Preparation:

Peel the avocado and cut in half. Remove the pit and cut into chunks. Add it to the bowl with melon and set aside.

Peel the lime and cut lengthwise in half. Set aside.

Cut the honeydew melon lengthwise in half. Scoop out the seeds using a spoon. Cut the large wedges and peel them. Cut into small chunks and place in a bowl. Wrap the rest of the melon in a plastic foil and refrigerate.

Wash the mint leaves and soak in water for 5 minutes.

Now, process avocado, lime, honeydew melon, mint, and pineapple in a juicer. Transfer to serving glasses and serve immediately.

Enjoy!

Nutritional information per serving: Kcal: 321, Protein: 5.2g, Carbs: 46.8g, Fats: 22.6g

30.   Spinach Apple Juice

Ingredients:

½ cup spinach, torn

1 large Gala apple, cored

½ tsp ginger, ground

1 large cucumber

¼ cup fresh parsley, finely chopped

Preparation:

Rinse the spinach and parsley using a large colander. Drain and chop into small pieces. Set aside.

Core the apple and chop into bite-sized pieces. Place it in a medium bowl and set aside.

Chop the cucumber into thick slices and combine it with an apple.

Roughly chop the parsley and collard greens and combine it with remaining prepared ingredients.

Process all in a juicer until well juiced. Transfer to serving glasses and stir in the ginger.

Add some ice cubes or refrigerate before serving.

Enjoy!

Nutritional information per serving: Kcal: 96, Protein: 3.1g, Carbs: 28.7g, Fats: 1.2g

31.   Salted Tomato Asparagus Juice

Ingredients:

3 large tomatoes, chopped

1 cup asparagus, trimmed and chopped

4 large carrots,sliced

2 medium-sized zucchinis, peeled and chopped

¼ tsp salt

Preparation:

Wash the tomatoes and cut into quarters. Cut in a bowl to reserve the juices. Set aside.

Wash the carrots and cut into small pieces. Set aside.

Peel the zucchinis and remove the seeds. Cut into bite-sized chunks and set aside.

Wash the asparagus and remove the woody ends. Chop into small pieces and set aside.

Combine tomatoes, carrots, zucchinis, and asparagus in a juicer and process until juiced.

Transfer to serving glasses and add a little bit of milk to adjust the thickness of the juice. Stir in the salt.

Serve immediately.

Nutrition information per serving: Kcal: 92, Protein: 5.4g, Carbs: 27.3g, Fats: 0.9g

32. Ginger Pomegranate Juice

Ingredients:

1 tsp fresh ginger, freshly grated

½ cup pomegranate seeds

½ cup fresh kale, torn

1 large Granny Smith's apple, cored

1 tbsp agave nectar

Preparation:

Peel the ginger knob and grate. Fill up the measuring teaspoon and reserve the rest in the refrigerator.

Cut the top of the pomegranate fruit using a sharp knife. slice down to each of the white membranes inside of the fruit. Pop the seeds into a medium sized bowl.

Rinse the kale thoroughly. Drain and torn into small pieces. Set aside.

Wash the apple and remove the core. Cut into bite-sized pieces and set aside.

Process the pomegranate seeds, kale, and apple in a juicer until well juiced.

Transfer to serving glasses and stir in the ginger. Add some water to adjust the thickness and stir in the agave nectar.

Serve immediately.

Nutrition information per serving: Kcal: 194, Protein: 6.2g, Carbs: 54.2g, Fats: 2.4g

33.   Lemon Chia Juice

Ingredients:

1 whole lemon, peeled

3 tbsp chia seeds

1 large yellow bell pepper, seeded

1 large Red Delicious apple, cored

Preparation:

Peel the lemon and cut into quarters. Set aside.

Wash the bell pepper and cut into halves. Remove the seeds and chop into small pieces.

Wash the apple and remove the core. Cut into bite-sized pieces and set aside.

Combine bell pepper, apple, and lemon in a juicer. Process until juiced.

Transfer to serving glasses and stir in the chia seeds. Add 2-3 tablespoons of water and stir again.

Stir well and serve immediately..

Enjoy!

Nutrition information per serving: Kcal: 135, Protein: 4.2g, Carbs: 31.3g, Fats: 6.2g

34. Artichoke Spinach Juice

Ingredients:

1 cup artichoke, chopped

1 cup fresh spinach, torn

1 cup avocado, cubed

1 cup green cabbage, torn

¼ tsp ginger powder

Preparation:

Trim off the outer layers of the artichoke using a sharp paring knife. Cut into bite-sized pieces and fill the measuring cup. Reserve the rest for later.

Combine spinach and cabbage in a large colander. Wash thoroughly under cold running water. Drain and torn into small pieces. Set aside.

Peel the avocado and cut lengthwise in half. Remove the pit and cut into small cubes. Fill the measuring cup and reserve the rest in the refrigerator.

Now, combine artichoke, spinach, avocado, and cabbage in a juicer and process until juiced. Transfer to a serving glass and stir in the ginger powder.

Refrigerate for 10 minutes before serving.

Nutrition information per serving: Kcal: 282, Protein: 15.4g, Carbs: 42.6g, Fats: 23.2g

35.   Lemon Mango Juice

Ingredients:

2 whole lemons, peeled and halved

1 cup mango, chunked

1 whole grapefruit, peeled and wedged

1 small Red Delicious apple, cored

¼ tsp ginger, ground

1 tbsp agave nectar

Preparation:

Peel the lemons and cut each lengthwise in half. Set aside.

Peel the mango and cut into chunks. Fill the measuring cup and reserve the rest for later. Set aside.

Peel the grapefruit and divide into wedges. Cut each wedge in half and set aside.

Wash the apple and cut lengthwise in half. Remove the core and cut into bite-sized pieces. Set aside.

Now, combine lemon, mango, grapefruit, and apple in a juicer and process until juiced. Transfer to serving glasses and stir in the ginger, milk, and agave.

Add few ice cubes and serve immediately.

Enjoy!

Nutrition information per serving: Kcal: 155, Protein: 4.5g, Carbs: 23.8g, Fats: 1.8g

36.   Ginger Plum Juice

Ingredients:

1 whole plum, chopped

¼ tsp ginger, ground

1 cup cantaloupe, chopped

1 cup fresh mint, torn

1 large orange, peeled

Preparation:

Cut the cantaloupe in half. Scoop out the seeds and flesh. Cut and peel one large wedge. Chop into chunks and fill the measuring cup. Reserve the rest of the cantaloupe in a refrigerator.

Wash the mint thoroughly under cold running water. Torn into small pieces and set aside.

Peel the orange and divide into wedges. Cut each wedge in half and set aside.

Wash the plum and cut in half. Remove the pit and chop into small pieces. Set aside.

Now, combine plum, cantaloupe, mint, and orange in a

juicer and process until juiced. Transfer to a serving glass and stir in the ginger.

Serve immediately.

Nutrition information per serving: Kcal: 151, Protein: 4.4g, Carbs: 45.6g, Fats: 0.9g

37.   Sour Fuji Cinnamon Juice

Ingredients:

1 large Fuji apple, cored

1 whole lime, peeled

¼ tsp cinnamon, ground

1 cup watermelon, chopped

1 large banana, chopped

1 cup fresh mint, torn

Preparation:

Wash the apple and cut lengthwise in half. Remove the core and chop into bite-sized pieces. Set aside.

Peel the lime and cut lengthwise in half. Set aside.

Wash the mint thoroughly under cold running water. Drain and torn into small pieces. Set aside.

Cut the watermelon in half. Cut one large wedge and wrap the rest in a plastic foil and refrigerate. Peel the slice and cut into small cubes. Remove the pits and fill the measuring cup. Set aside.

Peel the banana and cut into small chunks. Set asid

Now, combine apple, lime, watermelon, banana, and mint in a juicer and process until juiced. Transfer to a serving glass and stir in the cinnamon.

Add some crushed ice and serve immediately.

Nutrition information per serving: Kcal: 236, Protein: 4.6g, Carbs: 66.4g, Fats: 1.1g

38.   Lemon Honey Juice

Ingredients:

1 whole lemon, peeled

1 tsp liquid honey

1 cup grapefruit, chopped

2 large oranges, peeled

¼ tsp of ginger, ground

Preparation:

Peel the lemon and cut into quarters. Set aside.

Peel the grapefruit and divide into wedges.. Cut each wedge in half and set aside.

Peel the oranges and divide into wedges. Set aside.

Wash the kale leaves and roughly chop it.

Now, process lemon,grapefruit, and oranges in a juicer. Transfer to serving glasses and add some water to adjust the thickness if needed. Stir in the liquid honey and ginger.

Serve immediately.

Nutrition information per serving: Kcal: 128, Protein: 7.3g, Carbs: 34.5g, Fats: 1.1g

39.   Orange Cinnamon Juice

Ingredients:

1 large orange, peeled

2 large carrots, sliced

1 cup fresh strawberries

2 large Granny Smith's apples, cored

¼ tsp cinnamon, ground

Preparation:

Peel the orange and divide into wedges. Set aside.

Wash carrots and cut into small pieces. Set aside.

Wash strawberries and cut them into halves. Set aside.

Wash apples and cut in half. Remove the core and cut into bite-sized pieces. Set aside.

Now, process orange, carrots, strawberries, and apples in a juicer. Transfer to the serving glasses and stir in the cinnamon. Optionally, add some water if needed.

Refrigerate for 15 minutes before serving.

Nutrition information per serving: Kcal: 104, Protein: 3.9g, Carbs: 31.2g, Fats: 1.1g

40.   Pomegranate Lime Juice

Ingredients:

1 cup pomegranate seeds

1 whole lime, peeled

1 small Granny Smith's apple, cored

1 cup blueberries

¼ tsp ginger, ground

2 oz water

Preparation:

Cut the top of the pomegranate fruit using a sharp paring knife. Slice down to each of the white membranes inside of the fruit. Pop the seeds into a measuring cup and set aside.

Peel the lime and cut lengthwise in half. Set aside.

Wash the apple and cut lengthwise in half. Remove the core and cut into bite-sized pieces and set aside.

Place the blueberries in a colander. Rinse well under cold running water and drain. Set aside.

Now, combine pomegranate seeds, lime, apple, and blueberries in a juicer and process until juiced. Transfer to a serving glass and stir in the ginger and water.

Refrigerate for 5 minutes before serving.

Enjoy!

Nutrition information per serving: Kcal: 206, Protein: 3.3g, Carbs: 61.1g, Fats: 1.8g

41.   Ginger Banana Juice

Ingredients:

1 banana, sliced

¼ tsp ginger powder

1 large celery stalk, chopped

1 small Granny Smith' apple, cored

1 tbsp aloe juice

1 cup cucumber, sliced

Preparation:

Peel the banana and cut into chunks. Set aside.

Wash the celery stalk and chop into bite-sized pieces. Set aside.

Wash the apple and cut in half. Remove the core and cut into bite-sized pieces. Set aside.

Wash the cucumber and cut into thin slices. Fill the measuring cup and reserve the rest for later. Set aside.

Now, combine banana, celery apple, and cucumber in a juicer. Process until juiced.

Transfer to a serving glass and stir in the aloe juice and ginger. Optionally, stir in some fresh lemon juice for a bitter taste.

Add some crushed ice and serve immediately.

Nutrition information per serving: Kcal: 174, Protein: 2.7g, Carbs: 50.3g, Fats: 0.8g

42.   Cucumber Zucchini Juice

Ingredients:

1 cup cucumber, sliced

1 small zucchini, chopped

1 cup watercress, chopped

1 cup parsnip, sliced

¼ tsp ginger, ground

1 oz water

Preparation:

Wash the watercress thoroughly under cold running water. Drain and chop into small pieces. Set aside.

Wash the cucumber and cut into thin slices. Fill the measuring cup and reserve the rest for later. Set aside.

Peel the zucchini and cut into thin slices. Set aside.

Wash the parsnip and trim off the green parts. slightly peel and cut into slices. Set side.

Now, combine watercress, cucumber, zucchini, and parsnip in a juicer and process until juiced. Transfer to a serving glass and stir in the water and ginger.

Add some ice and serve immediately.

Nutrition information per serving: Kcal: 100, Protein: 4.2g, Carbs: 29.9g, Fats: 0.9g

43.   Apple Ginger Juice

Ingredients:

1 small Golden Delicious apple, cored

1 small ginger knob, peeled and sliced

1 small pear, cored and chopped

1 medium-sized banana, peeled and chunked

1 cup fresh spinach, chopped

Preparation:

Wash the apple and cut in half. Remove the core and cut into bite-sized pieces. Set aside.

Peel the ginger knob and chop into small pieces. Set aside.

Wash the pear and remove the core. Cut into small pieces and set aside.

Peel the banana and cut into small chunks. Set aside.

Wash the spinach thoroughly under cold running water. Slightly drain and chop into small pieces. Set aside.

Now, combine apple, ginger, pear, banana, and spinach in a juicer and process until juiced. Transfer to a serving glass and refrigerate for 10-15 minutes before serving.

Enjoy!

Nutrition information per serving: Kcal: 247, Protein: 1.7g, Carbs: 73.9g, Fats: 1.7g

44.   Cantaloupe Mint Juice

Ingredients:

1 small Red Delicious apple, cored

1 large wedge of cantaloupe, chopped

1 cup fresh mint, chopped

1 cup mustard greens, chopped

1 oz milk

Preparation:

Cut the cantaloupe in half. Cut one large wedge and peel it. Cut into small pieces and set aside. Wrap the rest of the melon in a plastic foil and refrigerate for later.

Combine mint and mustard greens in a colander and wash thoroughly. Slightly drain and chop into small pieces. Set aside.

Wash the apple and cut lengthwise in half. Remove the core and cut into bite-sized pieces. Set aside.

Now, combine cantaloupe, mint, apple, and mustard greens in a juicer and process until juiced.

Transfer to a serving glass and stir in the water. Refrigerate for 10 minutes before serving.

Nutrition information per serving: Kcal: 152, Protein: 5.6g,

Carbs: 41.7g, Fats: 1.3g

45.   Orange Broccoli Juice

Ingredients:

1 large orange, peeled

1 cup broccoli, chopped

2 oz coconut water

1 whole lime, peeled and halved

1 cup cucumber, sliced

¼ tsp ginger, ground

Preparation:

Peel the orange and divide into wedges. Cut each wedge in half and set aside.

Wash the broccoli and trim off the outer leaves. Cut into small pieces and fill the measuring cup. Reserve the rest in the refrigerator.

Peel the lime and cut lengthwise in half. Set aside.

Wash the cucumber and cut into thin slices. Fill the measuring cup and reserve the rest for later.

Now, combine orange, broccoli, lime, and cucumber in a juicer and process until juiced. Transfer to a serving glass and stir in the coconut water and ginger. Add some ice and serve immediately.

Nutrition information per serving: Kcal: 106, Protein: 4.8g, Carbs: 33.3g, Fats: 0.6g

ADDITIONAL TITLES FROM THIS AUTHOR

70 Effective Meal Recipes to Prevent and Solve Being Overweight: Burn Fat Fast by Using Proper Dieting and Smart Nutrition

By Joe Correa CSN

48 Acne Solving Meal Recipes: The Fast and Natural Path to Fixing Your Acne Problems in Less Than 10 Days!

By Joe Correa CSN

41 Alzheimer's Preventing Meal Recipes: Reduce or Eliminate Your Alzheimer's Condition in 30 Days or Less!

By Joe Correa CSN

70 Effective Breast Cancer Meal Recipes: Prevent and Fight Breast Cancer with Smart Nutrition and Powerful Foods

By Joe Correa CSN